Back Pain

25 years of helping patients with Chronic Back Pain and Arthritis

Dr. Cary Yurkiw, DC

Copyright © 2019 Dr. Cary Yurkiw, DC
All rights reserved.
ISBN: 9781790913015

DEDICATION

I would like to thank God for the opportunity to write this book. I pray that it helps people with their Back Pain and Arthritis. I would also like to thank my family for their love and support.

Dr. Cary Yurkiw, DC

DISCLAIMER

This book is not medical advice for your specific back condition. Consult a health care professional for your specific condition because every person's health and body are different.

ACKNOWLEDGEMENTS

I would like to thank my wife Marcie, daughter Jaeda, son Colby, mother Fran, sister Tracy and mother in law Linda for reviewing several drafts of this book.

Dr. Cary Yurkiw, DC

Table of Contents

Dedication	....	i
Disclaimer	....	ii
Acknowledgements	....	iii
1 Introduction	....	1
2 How the Spine Works	....	4
3 Causes of Back Pain	....	9
4 Spinal Degeneration	....	11
5 Arthritis	....	14
6 Scoliosis	....	16
7 Spondylolisthesis	....	18
8 Spina Bifida	....	20
9 Discs	....	21
10 Stenosis	....	23
11 Origin of Chiropractic	....	25
12 Innate Intelligence	....	27
13 Subluxations	....	29
14 The Nervous System	....	31
15 Homeostasis	....	35
16 Inflammation	....	37
17 Scar Tissue	....	39
18 My Experience as a Patient	....	41
19 The Initial Visit and Adjustment	....	43
20 The Cracking Noise	....	46

22	Addiction and Dependency	....	51
23	Self Help	....	53
24	Posture is Important	....	55
25	The Relief Phase	....	57
26	Follow-Up	....	61
27	The First Progress Exam	....	66
28	Corrective Care	....	69
29	Lifestyle Changes	....	71
30	Nutrition is Important	....	75
31	Stress	....	82
32	Sleep	....	86
33	Mattress	....	89
34	Core Back Exercises	....	91
35	Relapses Can Happen	....	94
36	Weight Loss	....	97
37	Prevention and Maintenance	....	100
38	Conclusion	....	102
39	Help and Advice	....	104

1 Introduction

Back Pain and the common cold are the top reasons for doctor visits. Certainly, in my clinic over the past 25 years Back Pain is the #1 reason people come to see me. Back pain can be treated successfully even when previous attempts have failed and the condition is chronic and long standing.

I believe that each patient's circumstances are unique and need to be treated differently even though two patients may come in with the same condition. They may need different treatment plans to correct their back problem.

In this book I will share my experience treating different causes of back pain and my approach. Patients initially are taken through a complete history, examination, testing, and then diagnosed correctly. Then we begin the process of treatment which includes going through phases of care including Relief, Correction, and Maintenance.

Patients increasingly take responsibility for their health as the treatment progresses. I believe educating the patient is important for better self-care and to make better health decisions long term.

Patients also need to understand their symptoms and what their symptoms are telling them about their health condition. I know patients initially just want pain relief when they come to my clinic, but pain is just the tip of the iceberg. Pain is a clue that there is something else much deeper that the patient needs to pay attention to. And the sooner the patient pays attention to that pain and the underlying problem the better. The faster I can start working on back pain when it presents the better the chances of stopping future re-occurrences and spinal degeneration otherwise known as Osteoarthritis.

Back Pain can have far reaching effects on general health. The spine is the core of the body and problems in the spine can affect the nerve flow going through the spinal cord. Also muscles around the spine, discs between the bones, and nerves that come out of the spine are affected by poor posture and spinal misalignment. This can lead to many other health problems in the tissue and organs connected to the spine through the nerve roots.

A poorly aligned spinal segment, which Chiropractors call a subluxation, can interfere with the nerve flow and cause a variety of health conditions because the nerves are powerful. The nerves allow communication, energy and electricity to travel between the brain and every cell, organ and tissue in the body.

The spine plays an important role in protecting the spinal cord but also allows us to move, bend and twist. We depend on a healthy spine and nervous system to work, play sports, go for walks, garden and all the things we love to do. And we expect to do those activities long term and be pain free.

Back Pain and spinal decay can cause serious complications to a person's health and well-being. If the spinal health is poor, it can lead to disability over time. Disability can lead to loss of work, enjoyment in life, feeling down and depressed. Patients try to cope and often turn to self-medication. Some try to crack their own backs for relief. Some try different types of treatment only to have the pain come back again and get discouraged with the results. Some patients have given up on living a normal and healthy life.

But there is hope! Finding the cause and correcting it restores the patient's ability to live again! It allows the patient to work, do activities with loved ones, enjoy hobbies and stay active in sports.

This book details the average patient's journey in my clinic from chronic back pain to healing and wellness.

2 How the Spine Works

I think it is important for patients and the reader of this book to understand the basics of how the body works. We call the study of the way the body works physiology. When patients understand how the physiology works, how the body is structured and how it heals it lays the foundation for better self-care and better results long term.

The spine is composed of 24 bones called vertebra. At the bottom of the spine are two additional bones called the sacrum and coccyx which most people call their tailbone. There is a small percentage of people with an extra vertebra in the spine or one less, but it isn't that common. Sometimes a bone in the sacrum or tailbone area will not fuse properly to the other ones and the result will be an extra segment in the lumbar spine.

The low back is composed of 5 vertebrae. And they are numbered top down from 1-5. In the Lumbar Spine we refer to the segments at L1, 2, 3, 4, and 5. Similarly, the neck or cervical are numbered from top down C1, C2 all the way to C7. And in the mid back or Thoracic Spine there are 12 bones that are numbered from T1 to T12.

The normal curve of the Lumbar spine is called a lordosis from front to back and curves into the body. The curve is important because curves are more flexible than flat spines. I do see patients that come into the clinic with loss of the spinal curvature and it makes the patient's spine very stiff and rigid. It can also lead to early degenerative changes called Arthritis, Osteoarthritis or Spinal Degeneration because the physics of the spine changes. Instead of each vertebra contributing to shock absorption and spreading out the load of weight bearing over all the segments equally, the spine gets over worked in the area that is out of place and cannot handle it well.

If the patient has too much curve front to back in their spine it is called a hyper-lordosis or if there is too little it is called a hypo-lordosis.

If you look at the body from left to right the spine should be straight down the middle. But if it curves to the right or left, we call that a scoliosis. A scoliosis can affect multiple vertebrae in the spine and sometimes goes one way in one area of the spine and then the opposite way in another area. It is common to see an "S" shaped curve where the thoracic spine goes one way and the lumbar the other to offset each other and try to keep the body balanced.

Discs are large in volume and about 1/3 of the height of the bone itself and provide lots of space for the bones so they don't touch each other. The space between the bones are required for the nerves to come out from the spinal cord and travel through a nerve root to other areas of the body. This is how the brain communicates with the body and regulates the cells, tissues and organs in the body simultaneously resulting in a continual balance in the body called homeostasis. There are hundreds of nerve impulses per second going up and down the spinal cord. This makes the body very adaptable to changes in the internal and external environment because of the constant nerve control and monitoring by the brain and its connection to all the cells, tissues and organs in the body.

The body's internal ability to regulate and heal itself is called Innate. It is programmed in our DNA. It's amazing that when a sperm and egg come together the combined cell knows what to do to grow into a baby and make all the organs systems. One of the most important developments is the notochord which develops into the spine.

A good example of Innate is when you get a cut or a bruise the body begins a process of inflammation, repair and healing until the tissues are restored to the way they were prior to the trauma. Occasionally if the trauma is bad enough and the conditions are not right for the best healing process to occur the tissues will heal but may not be restored completely to the way they were before. The area may be left with some scar tissue.

The same healing process that you see on the outside of your body when you have a cut or a bruise, happens on the inside of your body in and around the spine. But patients can't see inside the body so it is more of a mystery because the patient cannot see the spine healing and must rely more on how they feel and what they are able to do with their backs.

The spine is like a "Breaker Panel" in your home. I love using this analogy with my patients because they can easily relate. If your toaster is not working, and the lights go out in the kitchen, then there is a bigger problem than just the individual items.

A person would go to the breaker panel and look for the one labelled "kitchen" and then turn it back on. In the body, for example, when someone comes into the clinic with symptoms like pain in their back and numbness in their leg, I go to the breaker panel in the body which is the spine. I look for the segments and nerve that is labelled the Sciatic in the L4 to S3 area and find the bone out of place that is causing the problem.

There is one nerve root on the left and one on the right between each segment in the spine. A shift in the spinal alignment can affect the nerve on one side of the spine, or the other side and, in some cases, both nerves depending on how the segment shifts out of place. The vertebra and spine move in a three-dimensional plane and there are many combinations of mis-alignments.

Dr. Daniel David Palmer was the founder of Chiropractic and his theory was based on cause and effect. If a bone was out of place it interfered with the nerve flow and the connection between the brain and the cells, tissues and organs in the body via the spinal cord and nerve roots.

If there was nerve interference, then the signals were weak between the brain and the body and that caused the body to function at a lower level. Symptoms would eventually develop as a warning sign that there was a problem in the area. Eventually more serious dysfunction, disease, weakness, tiredness and sickness would be the result.

At times patients disregard the early warning signs of back pain. They hope the pain will go away but re-occurrences become more frequent. Patients try to cope by self-medicating and at times try to crack their own back to get relief. Unfortunately, that doesn't work to correct the cause and is a bad idea for long term results.

The symptoms may go away for a while as the body tries to cope and adapt. But eventually the symptoms return repeatedly and then the spinal condition worsens causing disability which leads to the patient seeking medical help.

The first doctor visit may include an exam and tests but usually a pain killer, muscle relaxer, or anti-inflammatory are prescribed. If doctor visits become more frequent further testing may be indicated like MRI, CAT scan or nerve conduction tests. A referral to a surgeon may be recommended.

Patients often get discouraged with the short-term results and temporary relief from doctor and therapist visits. Patients may feel like giving up. They may start to believe that they must learn how to live with their condition long term.

But there may be a better solution and that is to find the cause of their pain and correct it before it's too late!

3 Causes of Back Pain

Most people come to see me after weeks or months of pain and it is often not their first occurrence. We call back pain that is long standing "chronic" in the clinic versus "acute" which is more recent. We know the longer the back pain has been there and the more re-occurrences the harder it is to treat because the spine and joints start to breakdown and wear out. This process is called degeneration, arthritis, or more specifically osteoarthritis.

When I first meet a patient and do their history, exam and testing I want to arrive at a diagnosis for their condition. The diagnosis describes the patient's condition and the structures involved. Some common diagnoses in the clinic include Spinal Sprain, Scoliosis, Spondylolisthesis, Herniated Disc, Arthritis, Facet Syndrome, Stenosis, and Nerve Entrapment to name a few. Sometimes the diagnosis will be more specific like Sciatica that describes the sciatic nerve getting pinched.

The first episode of back pain could have been an injury at work, playing sports, a car accident, or nothing significant at all. Sometimes it's something minor like bending down to pick something up off the floor and the patient's back goes out.

The pain eventually goes away without treatment as the body gets used to the mis-alignment but the patient's back never feels the same again. The area is now a weak spot that is susceptible to re-injury. Most people will use pain killers, anti- inflammatories, or muscle relaxers on subsequent occurrences to help cope with the pain and dysfunction. Sometimes they will miss time from work and just rest their back until the symptoms go away and the inflammation settles.

Often people refer to their condition as having a "bad back" and that they cannot do certain things anymore because of their bad back. Over time patients are less and less confident in their ability and start to restrict their activities. The back weakens when a patient does not use it as much. The old saying "if you don't use it you will lose it" applies to most back conditions.

Atrophy develops as the muscles and ligaments around the spine are used less. This creates a negative feedback loop that feeds off itself making the disability worse and the spine starts to wear out quicker because of its' lack of use. The spine needs movement and full function to be healthy.

4 Spinal Degeneration

I like to look at x-rays of the spine to determine if there is pathology, check for mis-alignments, and to determine how long the bones have been out of place. I can see degenerative changes in the spine on x-ray. I classify the stages of degeneration in the spine from normal to phase 4.

If the spine is out of place for months or years, the spinal degenerative process can progress and become extensive. Pain, inflammation and muscle spasms are the most common symptoms.

On x-ray I see the spine changing alignment first. The bones continue to have the right appearance and the disc spaces are well maintained. But the alignment is crooked. The spine is three dimensional so it can shift left to right, front to back, and tip up or down. The subluxations start to cause nerve tension and interference. The spinal cord and nerve roots can be thought of like a rope and when the spine has the normal alignment there is slack in the rope. But when the spine shifts the rope gets stretched and then it can narrow causing nerve impulses to become irregular.

If the poor alignment and posture continues the spine starts to break down because the soft tissues cannot handle the increased workload. The discs act like shock absorbers and they start to break down first because they are the most susceptible and the softest. Discs are more like jelly donuts and the bones are like bricks.

Some disc material may start to get squeezed into the front and back parts of the spine. Behind the disc is the spinal cord in the spinal canal. Disc material may start to squish into the canal and can cause pressure to develop on the Central Nervous System. The pressure can also develop on the nerve roots coming out of the sides of the spine.

If the spine and posture remain the same and are not corrected the spine will progress to phase 2 of spinal degeneration. In phase 2 the bones start to change shape from the poor mechanics of the spine. They are only so strong and if the physical forces overwhelm the integrity of the bone it needs to adapt and change shape. The shape of the bone becomes more horizontal than vertical losing height as part of the adaptation.

This process is a major contributor to people losing height over time because the bony material is displaced horizontally rather than vertically. Also, conditions like Osteoporosis weaken the bone and speed up the collapse of the vertebra.

Sometimes patients are confused about the words Osteoporosis and Osteoarthritis. Osteoporosis is a weakening of the bone and Osteoarthritis is degeneration and breakdown of the bone. They are two separate and unique conditions.

The space behind the spinal bones and discs is called the Spinal Canal. If material pushes in from the bones and discs getting squished, it is called Stenosis. This can affect the nerve flow in the Spinal Cord.

In phase 2 most doctors will tell patients that they see arthritic changes in the spine and the joints are starting to wear out. The viewer of the x-ray can see bone spurs starting to develop on the spinal bones as it wears down and adapts.

In phase 3 the spine continues to degenerate, and the function of the spine gets worse. There is much compensation of the muscles around the spine to guard the bones from shifting and putting more pressure on the nerves. The brain and body are now in protective mode and a negative cycle is well established.

As a Chiropractor it gets harder and harder to correct the spine as the stages progress. I like to stop the degeneration of the spine as soon as possible and reverse the effects on the body.

In phase 4 it is getting to be too late to help the patient where very little nerve flow is getting though the spine and the signals going to the organs and legs are minimized. Significant disability may be the result.

5 Arthritis

Arthritis is something that I see in the clinic every day. The word arthritis comes from "arthron" meaning joint and "itis" which is a disease.

Inflammation is a common reaction to the body being injured and needing repair. If joints are out of place and inflamed, they are prime candidates to break down and become arthritic over time.

There are different types of arthritis namely Osteoarthritis, Rheumatoid Arthritis, and Psoriatic Arthritis among the most common types.

If the joints in the spine are breaking down that is called Osteoarthritis. Some patients think that osteoarthritis is part of normal aging. That would mean that everyone who is 40, 50, or 60 would have a spine that looked the same on an x-ray. But that is not true. I see a wide variety of spinal conditions in people of all ages. I have seen 30-year-old spines look twice their age.

Age does play a part in the healing process as it takes longer to heal the older the patient is. There is more chance of injury the longer you live and with the slowing of the repair process, it will make it more difficult to recover. But all hope is not lost, and the patient does not have to learn how to live with their condition and accept that they are getting old because they have arthritis. Yet many patients have been told that they have Arthritis and they must learn how to live with their condition as it is a normal part of the aging process, but that is not true.

A good analogy for the arthritic process is the alignment of a car. If the car is out of alignment, then the tires and wheel joints will wear out unevenly. One side of the car will wear out much faster than the other side. The joints may begin to squeak and rub. The tires will wear bald on one side faster than the other.

This happened to me years ago when I took my car in for an oil change. After the oil change was complete the mechanic asked me to come over because he had something to show me. He showed me the wear and tear on the tires on the right compared to the left and said there must be an alignment issue with the car because the tread was far less on one side compared to the other.

6 Scoliosis

Scoliosis is a condition where the spine shifts left or right over multiple segments in the spine. Most often I see a "S" shaped curve in the spine with the mid back going one way and the low back the other way. Not as common is a "C" shaped curve in the spine with the spine only going one way.

There are many reasons for scoliosis but the most common is the patient that started to grow crooked in their early teenage years and kept growing more and more crooked during their teens. In more severe cases organ function can be affected because the chest cavity and abdomen can become twisted and compressed causing function to become limited.

Scoliosis changes the tissues around the spine because of the mis-alignments. On one side the ligaments shorten and the other side they get stretched to accommodate the position of the spinal bones. The muscles on one side of the spine stretch and on the other side it contracts. This causes weakness and imbalance in the muscles and can cause tension in the area of the spine that is affected. As an example, patients can turn one way but cannot turn the other way as far.

In the clinic I check the alignment of the head, shoulders, hips and legs to detect the overall posture of the body. When a patient has a scoliosis, posture is affected, and the body is not level. The untrained eye may not notice it, but to a Chiropractor the change to the postural levels are obvious.

Patients may notice the postural changes from scoliosis when one arm and leg are longer than the other because of the shift in the shoulders and hips attached to the spine. People have clues that they are unbalanced when they need to get their clothes tailored as one pant leg or sleeve length is shorter than the other.

7 Spondylolisthesis

Spondylolisthesis is a slippage of one vertebra forward on top of another inside the spine. Most often this happens at the last segment in the spine called L5, but it can happen in other areas as well.

When the back is put under a lot of strain like in some sports it can cause small fractures in the back part of the vertebra because it cannot deal with the extreme movements well. Think about a gymnast and how far back they can bend. As the spinal bone heals and adapts to the stress that is being put on it the vertebra grows and elongates and then can shift forward on top of another vertebra as an adaptation to the activity.

The slippage can distort the disc because it is attached between the bones and this causes the disc to bulge. More of a concern is that the disc material can squish into the spinal canal or forwards into the front of the spine.

The pushing backward of the disc material combined with the bone slipping forward can cause a narrowing of the canal where the spinal cord travels from the brain down to the body. The spinal cord is the main highway of communication in the body. Pressure on the spinal cord can causes a variety of symptoms because of the great amount of nerve pressure and interference that develops.

We grade Spondylolisthesis from grade 1-5. If the slippage of one vertebra on top of another is 0-25% we call that a grade 1, then 25-50% would be a grade 2, 50-75% would be grade 3, 75-100% is grade 4 and if the vertebra is right off the one below or over 100% it is a grade 5.

8 Spina Bifida

Spina Bifida is a common condition that we usually see on x-ray. Spinal Bifida Occulta is when the outer part of the bone in the spine does not close properly when it is developing. It can run in families and is associated with mothers who do not have enough folate in their diet. Pregnant moms need good nutrition for their babies to be healthy.

Most of the time Spinal Bifida Occulta goes unnoticed but there are more advanced forms called Meningocele and Myelomeningocele. If I find Spina Bifida on a patient's x-ray, I make sure I let the patient know immediately.

In cases like Spina Bifida Occulta I like to look at the x-rays and be aware of where the deformity is and work with the area safely and effectively.

9 Discs

The discs in the spine are like jelly donuts. They have a tougher outer layer and a fluid filled center. The outer fibers of the disc are ligamentous and attach strongly into the bones above and below via Sharpey's Fibers.

Discs work as shock absorbers in the spine. They cushion the impact of physical strain and compression on the body. Discs do not slip like some patient's believe. They are not like hockey pucks that slip between bones. They are well anchored and attached to the bones.

They can however bulge to one side when squished unevenly. If a person has a misalignment in the spine that can cause a disc to bulge. It would be like taking your hands and pressing on a jelly donut unevenly. If the disc is bulging and now the patient repeatedly twists, moves and bends the dough can stretch and tear and then the liquid could push into the dough. That would cause a fluid pocket in the dough.

If that went further over time the dough could continue to tear and the fluid move right through and out of the donut. That would leave the jelly donut with less volume and then the dough would squish together.

The problem with the above scenario is that the space between the bones is only so high and if the disc becomes irregular then the material can compress on one side and that can narrow the space for the nerve to come out of the spine. This can pinch or trap the nerve and cause pain and disability.

My goal is to catch a disc bulge as soon as possible. I then want to re-align the segments above and below the disc, so the disc material is more concentric, and the shape is restored.

10 Stenosis

Stenosis is narrowing of the spinal canal. Subluxations over a long period of time cause the soft tissues to start to degenerate first. Discs are softer than bones and they get squished and compressed before the bones are affected. When the disc gets squished the material pushes forward and backward. When it pushes back it starts to narrow the spinal canal.

The spinal canal is where the spinal cord travels through from the brain to the body. The spinal cord can get compressed and then it can short circuit. The spinal cord is the main nerve highway in the body, like an Interstate highway. Signals will not be able to get through from the brain to the body.

Spinal Stenosis is the result of degeneration and arthritic changes in the spine from long-standing subluxation and damage to the discs and vertebrae. As the spine remains out of place for a long period of time the bones start to degenerate. They break down and flatten pushing the bony material forward and backward. This changes the shape of the bones to more of rectangular shape than square. I see this on x-rays.

The bone material can start to push into the canal as well building up pressure and interfering with nerve flow in the spinal cord. This can decrease the signal and power going from the brain down the spinal cord to the body in the main highway of the spine.

If the patient's spinal alignment and health is not corrected and, if the process continues, the interference can become more serious and the disability can progress. Most notably a patient's legs can get weak from poor nerve flow and energy. Eventually the patient may need a cane, walker or wheelchair because of the nerve flow to the muscles in the legs get so weak. I want to prevent the stages of degeneration from progressing because the symptoms and disability can become more severe and wide ranging.

Now that the reader knows more about the spine and different conditions that affect the spine let's turn to the Origin of Chiropractic and how I apply that to various back conditions in the clinic.

11 Origin of Chiropractic

When I went to Chiropractic College, I was taught the history of Chiropractic and the origin of the profession. Chiropractic is unique compared to other professions in its' treatment of back pain because of its' origin and philosophy.

Chiropractic started over 100 years ago when Dr. Palmer was studying how the body worked and healed. A janitor in his building put a bone out of place in his neck causing his hearing to be reduced.

Dr. Palmer knew that there were nerve connections between the brain and the organs through the spine. The body could heal itself if there was no nerve interference. The brain and body have an innate ability to keep a balance called Homeostasis in the body. If a bone is out of place it affects the nerve flow to the tissues and organs. If the janitor's spine was put back in place, then the hearing would be restored. It was a cause and effect relationship.

Dr. Palmer adjusted the bone that was out of place. The reader probably anticipates what happened when Dr. Palmer did the adjustment. The janitor's hearing improved. A profession was born, based on the principle that a properly aligned spine would allow the proper nerve flow to get through but one that was out of alignment would interfere with the nerve flow.

Other health care professions use some of the same techniques as Chiropractors, like manipulation. But the reason why Chiropractors do the adjustment is important and it is what makes Chiropractic unique. Spinal adjustments have been around for millennia. Only in the last 100 years has the spine been studied more intensely as the art, philosophy, and science of Chiropractic has progressed and evolved to restore health in the body.

12 Innate Intelligence

Innate intelligence is the inborn ability for the body to heal. I have learned a lot more about DNA in the past 20-30 years as more research is done especially in the field of genetics.

People are now more interested in natural healing and organics. Many people are eating better and are more conscious of chemicals and toxins in their food.

I think the body's ability to heal or Innate Intelligence was programmed in our DNA when God made us. Every person has the Innate Intelligence to heal no matter what age the person is. The field of genetics is becoming more and more advanced as genomes are mapped, and certain genetic abnormalities are linked to a pre-disposition to certain health problems.

Inside the genes are protein sequences that make us unique as a species and unique from one individual to another. The genes express themselves and cause our eyes and hair to be a certain color. The variation can be a fraction of a percentage that separates us from other mammals. And even more finite is the difference between one person and another.

Our genetic expression can be modified by epigenes. Epigenes are genetic modifiers that attach themselves to the genes so that the expression of the gene is altered. Certain circumstances in a person's life or even a group of people can lead to modification to a person's genetic expression. For example, if there were a famine and people needed to adapt to having no food the epigenes would work to modify the genetic expression to adapt to the famine.

Genes and DNA are important for our health. I think we have underestimated our bodies ability to heal but are now becoming more aware of how we can tap into that healing potential.

I think Dr. Palmer and the Chiropractic profession were ahead of their time with that belief over 100 years ago. I think allowing the innate intelligence to do its work and the brain to connect more strongly with the body via an aligned spinal column has so much potential to be studied and applied to many health conditions.

13 Subluxations

Subluxations are bones that go out of place and affect nerve flow. Dr. Palmer and his students believed that people get subluxations from physical force, toxins and auto suggestion. Over 100 years later our language has changed and so has the research on subluxations.

Today the way that translates is physical forces, toxins, and stress will cause subluxations. In the clinic I am even more specific with patients explaining how their specific history resulted in subluxations in their spine.

People have had car accidents, work injuries, and poor posture that have resulted in subluxations. A poor diet, alcohol, drugs, and bad habits like smoking can cause toxins to build up in the body. Also, contamination of our drinking water and preservatives in our food can cause heavy metals and other unwanted toxins to enter our system. A toxic body will not be a good environment for healing.

Stress is now being acknowledged as a major contributor to poor health as well. Bad stress over a long period of time can be toxic to our system, create tension and cause subluxations.

Dr. Cary Yurkiw, DC

14 The Nervous System

The nervous system is composed of 3 main parts. The signals go from the brain down the spinal cord to the tissue and organs via motor nerves. The signals come back from the body to the brain from the tissues and organs through the spine via sensory nerves. And the third system that is sometimes overlooked by health care professionals is the Autonomic Nervous System (ANS) which I believe is as important or more important than the motor and sensory nerves.

Nerves are coated with insulation around them called myelin to keep the electricity in the nerve, so it does not jump out like in like Multiple Sclerosis. The reader can think of nerves like extension cords that you may use in your home or yard. The reader can also think of nerves like internet cables that connect computers to a main server.

These sensory nerves communicate changes in the body to the brain using receptors. There are several receptors or sensors in the body that are highly aware of changes in the tissues. Some examples of receptors being activated would be changes in temperature in the body. Other types of nerves are sensitive to stretch and movement. Some receptors are sensitive to pressure changes. And some receptors are aware of chemical changes in the tissues.

And the sensors are much like the ones in your car, sending signals to the dashboard in your car detecting what is going on inside and out of the car.

The brain needs to know what is always happening in the body. There are signals traveling up and down the spinal cord at several times a second from each cell, tissue and organ to the brain. That is a lot of information to process at one time! But it is much like a fast and powerful computer.

The ANS is a system of nerves that come out of the spine and travels to each organ and tissue in the body. The ANS is interesting and important because it is composed of two sets of nerves that come out of different areas of the spine, connect to each organ in the body, and have the opposite effect on one another.

The ANS helps to keep the right tone in the body. This is important because the body needs the right tone to be responsive to changes in the internal and external environment. Not too much tension and not too little. Just the right amount for the organ to do its work as efficiently as possible.

The ANS is composed of sympathetic and parasympathetic nervous systems. The parasympathetic nerves come out of the top and bottom of the spine and go to all the tissue and organs in the body. The sympathetic nerves come out of the middle part of the spine and travel to the same tissues and organs in the body.

The area of subluxation is important because a subluxation in the mid back can affect the organs much differently than a low back subluxation. The two types of nerves in the ANS offset each other as one is stimulating the organ and the other relaxes and calms the organ. Both are required to balance the organ function and maintain the homeostasis in the body.

I do see disorders in the body caused by subluxations that affect just the sympathetic or parasympathetic nerves but not both. If the subluxation is in the middle part of the spine it blocks the flow of the sympathetic nerves to the organ. If the subluxation is at the top or bottom of the spine it blocks the parasympathetic nerve flow to the organ.

A typical example of irregular nerve flow to an organ that I see in the clinic is a patient with a subluxation in their lower spine affecting the nerve flow down the sciatic nerve but also the parasympathetic nerve flow to the organs in abdomen. Now the digestive system has too much sympathetic nerve flow but not enough parasympathetic. This causes an imbalance in the tone of the organ and can lead to decreased activity of the muscles in the intestines.

The sympathetic nerve flow slows down the digestive system but the parasympathetic speeds it up. The result can be constipation as the food moves through slowly and starts to irritate the intestinal lining. Also, gas and cramps are possible from the muscle tension and slow movement. Adjusting the spine to reset the nerve flow is important to re-balance the organ function so that the digestive system can work normally again.

This is one example of how one area of the spine can affect one organ system because of a lack of nerve flow. Keep in mind that all the organ systems in the body are connected to the spine though the nervous system. Too much or too little tone in the lungs, stomach or heart can cause increased or decreased tension in these organs leading to a variety of symptoms and health conditions.

Dr. Cary Yurkiw, DC

15 Homeostasis

Homeostasis is the process of the body establishing an equilibrium or balance between the different organs and systems. This is seen in the structure when one area shifts one way in the spine and then another area shifts the other way to compensate. Homeostasis is also present when the physiology of the body adapts and balances due to changes inside the body and out. When it is cold or hot outside the body changes to adapt.

When there is a subluxation and mis-alignment in the spine the body shifts to compensate. These changes are present structurally but also physiologically or functionally as well. Swelling, muscle spasm, ligament tension, nerve and blood flow are all affected in an area that is out of place.

The brain will do its best to optimize the changes in the body. The goal is to keep the body functioning to the highest level. With subluxations present that may mean the body is now only functioning 90% instead of 100%. If there is more subluxation that may decrease to 80% and so on.

Homeostasis is a constant equilibrium or balance between body parts and processes. It is a wonderful innate mechanism that we are born with and don't have to think about.

There are so many signals going from the body to the brain each second that it makes homeostasis possible. Changes in multiple areas of the body can be made in fractions of a second with proper nerve flow relaxing one area and exciting another area.

Homeostasis allows a person to be in harmony with the internal and external environment. There is compensation and re-compensation happening all the time in the body's physiology. The nervous system and spinal cord make this possible with lightning fast communication between the cells in one area of the body with another.

One change in the body can set off a reaction in several areas. In this way Chiropractic is a catalyst to make positive changes in the body by improving alignment and communication between the body parts allowing the innate homeostatic process to be maximized.

16 Inflammation

Inflammation is good for the healing process in the body. Patients often come in and think they need to take an anti-inflammatory as they think inflammation is bad. Inflammation is necessary for the tissues to heal and inflammation provides the right natural chemicals for healing to take place. The first step is inflammation for protection against further damage to the tissues. Next inflammation provides the right clotting factors for the tissues to stop bleeding if there is trauma. Next scar tissue starts to develop to patch up the area as the inflammatory response continues.

I generally tell my patients that the inflammation is there for a reason. If the patient can put up with the temporary discomfort from the inflammation which is a tender, red and hot area then that is best as the body will heal the quickest with its' natural processes taking place.

If a patient interferes with the inflammatory response it can slow the healing down. Rarely does inflammation progress to a serious or life-threatening condition.

Dr. Cary Yurkiw, DC

17 Scar Tissue

Scar tissue is a natural way for the body to heal an injured area. The tissue gets laid down in an irregular matrix to patch up an area. Scar tissue can develop on the outside of the body like on the skin. It can develop on the inside of the body around the spine. Scar tissue can happen in all parts of the body.

If there has been a severe trauma like a car accident or work injury, I like to give the scar tissue a few days to set up and to stabilize the area. The area may be stiff, swollen and weak.

After a few days I like to begin the healing process and get active with treatment. The scar tissue is still fresh, and I can make the greatest change before its irregular pattern sets up for too long.

The care must be gentle and metered so that the stability and integrity of the joints are maintained as the tissue is rehabilitated.

Careful follow up is important to do a little each day and see how the body is responding. This starts to work the scar tissue into more functional tissue. This allows the body to be more flexible and change the alignment and range of motion in the process.

I like to get the patient involved in stretching and exercise to help the process along. Together, the patient and I can make the most change to restore the tissue back to the way it was before the injury.

I am a big advocate of seeing a doctor as soon as possible after injury. It is easier to work with a fresh injury and scar tissue than a chronic condition that has existed for a long time.

18 My Experience as a Patient

I began seeing a Chiropractor when I was a young teenager for my knee pain. At times I had hip pain that felt like a sharp pinch in my low back off to the side. Our family doctor kept telling my parents that my knee pain was due to growing pains. I was playing hockey and active in other sports at school and had excruciating pain if I fell on my knees or bumped them. I couldn't walk at times the pain was so bad! Occasionally I had sacroiliac pain as well which felt like my hip had gone out. My father heard of a Chiropractor in our area that had many good reviews from people in our church and community.

He took me to the Chiropractor who did a history, examined my knees, and did x-rays. When my father and I returned for the next visit he explained that the bones in my knees were growing too fast, the muscles and tendons were too short, and that bones were separating in my knees. There was inflammation in my knees, and I had pain because of the process of re-injury and attempted repair to the tissues around my knees as this bad cycle continued.

He also explained that Chiropractic was a full body approach and he would work on my knees, hips, and spine to balance my posture and improve the nerve flow so my knees could heal properly.

I must admit that initially I was scared the treatments would hurt. The Chiropractor asked me to come in three times a week to start. I went to see him for months as the treatments decreased in frequency. As the treatment progressed the knee pain became less and less. I became stronger and could do more. My level of play in sports like hockey improved dramatically. I went from a low level of play in Tier 4 to a higher level eventually getting to Tier 1.

I had the desire to play at a higher level, but my physical condition and limitation was holding me back. Chiropractic allowed me to overcome the disability. I became more confident in my abilities. That really changed my life and made me think that I wanted to become a Chiropractor in the future. If I could help people, the way my Chiropractor helped me, that's what I wanted to do.

19 The Initial Visit and Adjustment

I have always focused extra time and attention at the beginning of care when I meet the patient for the first time. I want to get the best history, exam, and accurate diagnosis to have a good starting point for the patient care. Sometimes the patient requires extra tests, like x-rays, to view the alignment and condition of the spine and to rule out any pathology. Pathology can be a fracture, tumor, or other condition in the spine that would need urgent care at a hospital.

Putting all the information together from the patient history, examination, and any tests I determine a diagnosis for the patient's condition. Then I want to communicate this diagnosis to the patient before I start care and let the patient know what to expect going forward and between the sessions.

The first adjustment is my favorite one, because doing the adjustment usually brings so much relief for the patient. It is the first positive change to the area in a long time. It stops the negative feedback loop that is well established.

A small positive change is encouraging to the patient. I think it is a combination of pain relief and the ability to do more that brings hope and optimism back to the patient. Hope is so powerful for the patient because it is a small spark in their lives that can lead to more profound change.

I don't want to do too much on the first few sessions that would overwhelm the patient's body and make it difficult to monitor the changes in the area. I like to be specific with adjustments at the root of the cause. I like to determine the rate of healing and estimate how long it will take the patient to recover.

I also do not want to complicate the treatment by asking the patient to do more than just rest and enjoy the relief in the first few visits. If they have been doing certain things to help them with the pain, I tell them to continue for now because the pain will only be temporary. As the cause of the problem is corrected the pain subsides and the patient will not need to continue to take pain killers.

I also tell patients not to start anything new, so they don't complicate the healing process. Sometimes I find patients getting ambitious as they start to feel better and want to do a lot all at once. I want the treatment to progress like a good controlled experiment where one variable is changed at a time while the others remain constant.

The three phases of care I recommend in the clinic are Relief, Correction and Prevention. A care plan may start with 3 sessions a week for Relief, then progress to 2 sessions a week in Correction and then down to 1 session a week to Maintain and to Prevent re-occurrences. This process can take weeks to months to accomplish depending on how long it took to get that way and the patient's history, current lifestyle and pace of healing.

I also warn the patient that healing progresses like a sine wave. It fluctuates up and down as it trends upward. It is like two steps forward and one step back. Occasionally we have a patient that takes a step back after the first session before they go two steps forward, so I like to make patients aware of the potential for this to happen. Adjustments change the alignment in the area and the body reacts to the change.

20 The Cracking Noise

The cracking noise you hear in your joints when doing a manual or hands on adjustment is called cavitation. Cavitation is produced when the volume of the disc space is increased and the fluid and gas shifts in the capsule to one area causing a pressure change. The pop is not significant to the treatment outcome but sometimes patients associate the pop as a "good adjustment" if they do not understand what produced the pop or why we did that.

I like to educate patients about adjustments and how the body works so they understand that moving the bones in the spine into the right place produces relief and restores function. There are some techniques that do not produce a popping noise but are just as effective as ones that do. For example, an instrument adjustment does not produce a cracking noise, but it does move the bone and is just as successful as a hands-on adjustment.

I use a technique that pops up one piece of the table to then drop down as I do the adjustment and most of the time there is no noise from the joint when that is done but it is very affective.

There is another sound in the joints called crepitus which is different. It is more like a crackling noise when you move a body part. Crepitus is not significant, and I tell patients not to worry about the sound. Checking the underlying alignment and function is important but not the sound.

Bones can sometimes rub over bones and cause a noise when you move. This happens quite often in the scapula or shoulder blade area when the scapula glides over the ribs. Sometimes patients are concerned about this noise and will often demonstrate this movement for me causing the noise to be reproduced. I tell them not to worry about that but do not try to reproduce the sound as the friction can lead to irritation and then inflammation can develop causing the area to become uncomfortable.

Poor posture can lead to poor mechanics in an area. Slouching is a major cause of the scapula being pulled forward on the ribs. Then the ribs can start to rub against the scapula. To correct this, I work on the alignment and posture with the patient so that the body parts are in place and have lots of room to move, relieving any points of friction and sounds that may develop because of that.

The two noises I described above are much different from the sounds when you break a bone. If you have ever broken a bone the sound made from a bone breaking is much different than a crack or pop. It is more like a snap and totally different from the sounds described above.

Another sound that is common is a "clunking" sound that severely arthritic patients experience. The clunk is from instability in the joint and sounds terrible. Luckily, I don't have too many patients progress to the latter stages of Osteoarthritis when the clunking sound happens.

Dr. Cary Yurkiw, DC

21 Don't Crack Your Back!

This is a good time to talk about cracking your own back. Don't do it! It may feel better temporarily from the endorphin release associated with the crack but that only helps the pain for about 20 minutes or so. If you keep doing that just for the endorphin release, then you will become dependent on that chemical release in the body to feel good, but the bones are not getting re-aligned in the right place to correct the problem. You need a professional to do that for you. Even Chiropractors need Chiropractic care when they have mis-alignments and subluxations in their body!

Don't crack your back also applies to any joint in the body including your knuckles and neck which seem to be the other areas that people like to crack on their own, but it can lead to instability and re-enforcement of the poor position of the bones. Also, the compression from doing the adjustment wrong can cause damage to the joint and cartilage eventually. I think that is why your grandma may have told you not to crack your knuckles as you will get arthritis. It is from doing the adjustments wrong when the body may not need it. You may be compressing the joints causing trauma and begin the arthritic process. The joint may be in place and no adjustment is necessary.

I remember my first year in Chiropractic College and having a shoulder problem called Rotator Cuff from lifting weights in the gym. The weightlifting was pinching the tendon in my shoulder causing pain lifting my arm over my head. Some of the pain radiated up into my neck area. If I slept on my shoulder at night the pain in my shoulder woke me up. I was losing some sleep at night because of the pain.

I went to the clinic at the school to get help. The doctors and clinicians there told me that they would help to correct the Rotator Cuff problem, but I needed to stop cracking my neck and back. It was a bad habit that I developed over time to cope with the pain and achy feeling in my joints.

It took a lot of will power to resist cracking my neck at the beginning of care but as I got adjustments the relief became noticeable and I started to feel better and better. It became easier and easier to not crack my own joints until eventually I didn't do it at all.

22 Addiction and Dependency

Patients can become addicted to pain killers if they have had back pain for a long period of time and need stronger and stronger meds for their pain. Patients are given stronger drugs like narcotics at times that become addictive. Patients do start to depend on the drugs to feel good and sometimes take too many or want to get more before they can get their next prescription.

Sometimes people turn to alcohol and street drugs to help with their pain. Just dealing with the symptoms without correcting the underlying cause will lead to temporary relief and dependency on the drugs. The only way to get rid of the pain completely and long term is to correct the underlying cause. Pain is only a symptom warning the patient that something underneath needs attention.

Both addictions and time lost from work cost our economy a lot of money every year. Treating people with natural methods are increasingly seen as cost affective compared to the down time and cost to treat people addicted to drugs or not at work because of their back pain.

Today addiction is a big problem in our society and governments are looking for ways to get rid of pain more naturally. There are more natural products on the market now to help with the pain. Also, there is much more interest in Chiropractic as a result because it corrects the cause of back pain naturally.

23 Self Help

Patients often ask me, "What can I do to help?" Some patients are more eager than others to be involved. I like to see a patient that is highly motivated but not trying to make too many changes all at once especially early in care that could complicate the healing process. In the first few weeks it is a critical time to get the patient feeling better, start a positive cycle of healing, and follow up closely.

I have found that patients that want to make too many changes to their lifestyle early in care can complicate the recovery which makes monitoring the results confusing both for the patient and for me. Also making too much change to a patient's lifestyle at once can lead to failure as the right support systems are not in place for consistent and long-lasting change.

I like to let the first few adjustments take affect and see how the patient's body responds to the care. I like to monitor the pace of healing so I can give the patient a good estimate of how long the care will take when I make my recommendations in a Care Plan.

I like to keep it simple with one or two adjustments on the first session and keep the adjustments light and specific. Once I get to know the patient's body better, I can increase the intensity of the adjustments depending on what their body can handle.

I often tell patients to continue doing what they have been doing before they started care as long as it is not doing any harm. The only change I want to make is the adjustment to the spine. I don't want the patient to start anything new as well because the body could get overwhelmed with too much change all at once.

The opposite can be true as well and patients start to feel good with the care in the clinic and they don't want to do anything but come for the adjustments. Long term that is not good because they are relying too much on the work I am doing in the clinic and not on making changes at home that will support long lasting results. These changes at home are critical to support and to maintain the corrective work we are doing in the clinic.

I don't want patients to just rely on the Chiropractic adjustments for their relief but really correct the cause of their problem and long term take responsibility for their health.

There is plenty of time in the coming weeks of care to get involved and make lifestyle changes for patients. Changes to a patient's routine and lifestyle can take time and be difficult. Old routines are hard to break, and new ones can take much effort to establish and support.

24 Posture Is Important

Posture is important. If patients want better function and alignment of their back, then it is important to focus on posture. If you look at the spine left to right, it should be straight down the middle. But if you look at the spine the front to back it should have 4 curves that intersect a plum line drawn straight down the side of the body.

From front to back the most common mis-alignment that I see is the head forward in a "text neck" position and which flattens the upper forward cervical curve in the spine and then that causes an increased curve in the upper back that looks like a more rounded back with a bone sticking out where the neck and shoulders meet.

If the poor posture continues, I see the spine degenerating and wearing out faster than it should which is called Arthritis. People can appear to be stiff and have a forward leaning posture.

The changes in alignment cause discs to get squished on one side of the spine and for that side to wear out faster than the other as we discussed in the Arthritis chapter. The wear and tear on the spine are called degeneration and can be seen on x-ray. I want to do my best to correct the poor posture for the patient.

I will give patients postural exercises during care and tips on checking their alignment. They can look in a mirror and check the landmarks in the body being the level of their head, shoulders, hips and feet. Also, I give them quick postural resets that they can do at work or at home like pulling their shoulder blades down to reset the upper ribcage and get the head back in alignment with the shoulder.

Posture can also be affected by the quality of the bones. If the bones lose calcium, then they can become weak. At the start this process is called Osteopenia but if it progresses then it is called Osteoporosis.

This makes the bones brittle and they can start to compress and collapse more in the front part of the spine than the back part of the spine. The forward compression causes the bones to look more wedge shaped over time instead of square. This causes the back to round more excessively in the mid back and the back to appear arched.

I have seen many patients with Osteopenia and Osteoporosis over the years. My goal is to correct the patients posture and give them advice on how to strengthen their bones through their diet and increase their activity levels to make the bones stronger.

25 Relief Phase

The body begins trying to heal shortly after an injury occurs. This could be a major trauma, or it could be smaller micro traumas over time. If a bone shifts in your back immediately the brain starts to send signals to compensate for the shift. The vertebra above and below may go the other way to offset the subluxation or mis alignment. Muscles will start to tighten to protect and support the injured area.

Inflammation is the first step toward healing. Inflammation carries the chemicals needed for the area to heal. Inflammation starts a chemical chain reaction to contain the trauma and initiate the healing process.

Nerves are pinched and they throb and become very painful letting the patient know there is a problem in the area and the patient needs to pay attention to it. There is only so much room for the inflammation in the spine and sometimes pressure can build up causing compression on the tissues in the area.

Changes to the joint and surrounding area can affect the receptors located in the tissue. There are pain receptors called nociceptors and movement ones like mechanoreceptors in the tissues around the joint in your back.

The nerve endings are very sensitive to chemical changes. When inflammation and other irritants are present in the tissue the nerve endings send signals to the brain which results in the feeling of pain.

The mechanoreceptors are more powerful than the nociceptors and can block the pain signal where the two signals meet at the synapse. It's like two roads coming together but the mechanoreceptor signal gets to go first.

This is significant because I can use that in the clinic to get patients moving more and blocking the pain pathways early in care. The adjustments start a positive cycle of less pain, more movement, better alignment, and get the patient more active which helps with the next spinal adjustment because there is less tension in the area. The brain is not guarding the area as tightly as the position and function of the spine improves.

Most people just want to get rid of the pain when they first come to the clinic, but the problem is often much deeper than the pain. Pain is just the tip of the iceberg. And the cause is what is below the surface. It's important to address the underlying cause because the problem cannot be corrected unless the underlying cause is corrected.

The Relief Phase can take weeks to months. There are many factors that determine how long it will take including how long the problem has been there and the patient's current lifestyle in this phase. I don't want to just get some relief for the patient and take a few steps toward correction but then stop and let the symptoms come back again. If correction does not happen then the pain can come back again, and the inflammation may continue to irritate the area as it increases.

Often the body is in "protective" mode when it is in pain. The brain senses the pain and does not want any more pressure on the nerves. The brain must maintain communication with the body. Initially the body can be very guarded and stiff. It can be hard to adjust. It's protective of its' position and does not want to let go.

I find patients psychologically guarded as well because of the pain and the fear of more pain with work being done on the area. The speed of the adjustment is important and what overcomes the tension. Patients will often apologize and say they are sorry for tensing up, but I tell them not to worry it is the speed and not the force that makes an adjustment successful.

Sometimes moving the bone even a fraction of an inch can produce good results when the body is so locked up. I think the adjustments also gives the brain the confidence to let go a little bit. Now that the spinal segment has moved and there has not been a considerable increase in pain, the brain feels more confident to let go in the new position. The brain sends a signal to the muscles in the area around the spine to let go, release some tension to allow more movement.

This is really the start of the healing process. Initially inflammation is present but if the alignment and movement of the spine do not change then the inflammation will continue to go on forever trying to heal the underlying tissue which is dysfunctional. The adjustments are positive for the body. More nerve flow can get through and the signal is now stronger from the brain to the cells, tissues and organs.

The patients usually notice immediate relief. The adjustments feel good when they are done, and the worst part of care is over which is the fear of the first adjustment and the potential pain associated with it.

I believe that if more people knew how good adjustments did feel then I think they would try Chiropractic a lot sooner. When the adjustment is done it's like a sliver that has been pulled out of your finger. The patient feels great relief! And then the inflammation can do its job and heal the tissues.

The next step in care is the Corrective Care phase. Retraining the spine and posture to be in the right place long term. The body does tend to want to return to the old alignment especially if it has been that way for a long time. But following up with adjustments allows the process to continue. I like to keep the visits close together at the start of care so the patient can heal faster.

26 Follow-Up

After the first adjustment the patient usually starts to feel better. They leave the clinic knowing something good has happened. They go home and have a good sleep. But when they wake up in the morning, they feel sore again.

Swelling usually accumulates overnight when a person is not moving around very much. The inactivity also allows the nociceptors to send signals to the brain and the mechanoreceptors are not that active to inhibit pain signals from getting to the brain.

People feel worse in the morning compared to when they went to bed because of the increased swelling and inactivity. But the swelling will dissipate again as the person gets moving.

I generally schedule a new patient to come back the next day because I want to check on them and see what the alignment and pain level is like. I want to give them the best care possible and close follow up is essential.

I want to check the position of the bone and see how much the tissues have changed. Is the bone in the same position that I left it, or has it regressed trying to go back to the old position?

Patients usually have questions and feedback for me, and I want to be available to answer them. I also want to move the process forward with another adjustment, so they feel even better. That will then move the bone 2 more steps forward toward the goal before it takes another step back the next day.

People often ask me at this time what should they be doing to help the process? Why does one area feel better, but another is sorer? Why does it feel better and then it feels like it is coming back again? There is shifting and compensation happening up and down the spine with the adjustments. The body works as a unit so when one area is getting adjusted the other areas shifts to adapt.

If the patient is icing their back for relief, I will suggest they continue to do that. Whatever the patient is doing to help relieve the pain right now will help. Some people prefer heat as it works better for them. I tell the patient to keep their self-care consistent at the beginning because the only changes that I want to make are adjustments to the spinal alignment.

Long term the patient will not need to ice and heat and will not need pain killers because the symptoms will reduce, and the inflammation will go down, and the body will be restored back to the way it should be.

As for bigger changes to the patient's self-care I like to keep those recommendations until the care has progressed to the first progress exam.

I like to prioritize the changes I suggest from most important to least. I usually get an idea of what is most important from the history and getting to know the patient during care.

I do the second adjustment and then continue to follow up closely giving the patient a plan for the next two weeks. I remind the patient that the symptoms will be up and down as the body responds to the adjustments. Some days will be better than others. The pain in the back may start to go away but another pain may develop like in the hip or upper back. It's all part of the process of the body adapting to the new alignment.

I may need to work on other areas of the spine as the treatment progresses because I find it helps the body to re-compensate quicker and the healing to go faster than just working on one spot. If I didn't do the adjustments in the others area of the spine that have shifted to compensate, it would take longer for the patients to heal.

Initially, I like to define the primary subluxation and then work on the secondary subluxations later in care. The most common adjustment I do in the low back is at the L5 vertebra with the Sacroiliac joints being the second most common followed by L4.

There are many major nerves coming out of the low back. The greatest being the sciatic nerve. The sciatic nerve is composed of 5 nerve roots. The nerve roots are big and come together to form one nerve that supplies nerve flow to three quarters of the leg. The roots come from L4, L5 and S1, S2, and S3. Some lumbar nerve roots and some sacral nerve roots make up the Sciatic Nerve. The Femoral nerve that supplies the nerve flow to the upper front part of the leg has its' origin at L2-4 a little higher up the spine than the sciatic nerve.

When a patient has certain symptoms in a certain location it is a clue as to what could be out of place. Therefore, doing a good history is important.

During follow up care sometimes it is tempting for patients that are feeling better between sessions to try and test the area to see what it can handle. I discourage patients from doing that because it could set the healing back a couple steps. There is only so much the new alignment and posture can handle and if it is overwhelmed with too much physical force it may shift and go back into protective mode setting the care back a couple steps or more. This may also delay the healing process.

I like to make a recommendation within the first 5 sessions to the patient, so they know what to expect. I include as much detail as I can for the Relief, Correction and Preventative phases of care. The Care Plan is like a road map for care. It takes into consideration the unique circumstances for the patient and what the expectation is going forward.

Progress exams and reports are important checks and balances for the patient care. It gives me an opportunity to compare the previous exam results to the current ones and then report to the patient where they are now in their care.

Are they ahead of schedule? Are the behind? Or is the patient right on track? I use postural pictures and draw on them so patients can see for themselves how they are progressing. Also, periodically I do follow up x-rays to compare the original to how the patient is doing now. X-rays are like the gold standard in imaging because I can see inside the body and compare the changes from the start to that point in care.

I take advantage at the time of the progress reports to discuss with patients the changes I am seeing and discuss what the patient can do to help themselves. This may include lifestyle changes, nutrition, diet, stress, sleep, stretches and exercises.

I have recently added phone consultations to some of the patients' care plans if I think more detailed instruction is necessary and follow up to make sure the patient is staying on track.

I find that weekly calls can really help patients along in their care and lead to faster and better results.

27 First Progress Exam

The first progress exam happens around the six-week mark into care. At this point I want to check in and see how the patient is progressing. I want to relay the findings to the patients and let them know what they can do to help themselves. It also gives me an opportunity to make changes to the Care Plan if I need to because the patient may be healing faster or slower than I expect.

I like to have patients fill in a form so I can better understand how the patient is doing subjectively. I want to do tests again to compare objectively how the patient is doing compared to the last exam. I also take postural pictures against a grid that has 1 cm squares that allow me to compare the patient's postural levels from exam to exam.

I check the range of motion to see how much change there is. Is the person moving better? Are they more flexible? Is there less tension in the musculature? What is the tone like around the spine? I do orthopedic and neurologic tests to compare findings, the diagnosis and treatment plan.

Postural pictures are great for the patient because they can see how their posture and alignment is changing for the better. It is very rewarding for the patient when they can see it for themselves.

Once I review the findings with the patient, I move onto my recommendation for the next 6 weeks. Is the recommendation the same as my initial care plan or does it need to change? And then I want to give them specific stretches to help loosen ligaments, muscles and discs on one side of the spine to help me to make faster progress in the clinic.

The specific spinal stretches are the opposite way to the way the patient is out of place. This allows faster changes to the spinal alignment. I recommend that patients do these specific exercises first thing in the morning for consistency and better results.

If patients leave the stretches until later in the day, they may not get them done as other activities come up that get in the way. This is especially true if the patient is starting to feel a lot better and feels that they do not need to do the stretches every day.   I remind patients that it is the underlying cause that we are correcting not just dealing with the superficial symptoms.

If the stretches are getting too easy, I tell the patients to increase the amount.   Initially I will give the patients a recommendation of 15 repetitions but if that gets too easy, I tell patients to go to 2 sets of 15 repetitions that will be 30 reps total. If the patient gets to the point where 30 is too easy, I will recommend 3 sets of 15 or 45 repetitions. I will continue like that during care until the patient reaches 15 sets of 15 repetitions or 225 total repetitions and then they should keep doing the maximum.

I do give the patient sheets to take home that give them clear instructions on which directions to do the stretches.

I also ask them to record the number of sets and reps on the sheets.

Occasionally I have patients that want to do the stretches the other direction than the way the sheets say because they are feeling better. I advise them against that because at this point it would reinforce the imbalance that is already present in the spine.

28 Corrective Care

Corrective Care is the phase of care that I think makes the biggest difference for the patient long term. The patient is already feeling better and their alignment and posture is changing. Now I can begin to get the patient more involved in their care. I can give the patient more responsibility and reduce the frequency of the sessions.

Not everyone wants to go through the corrective process and take on more responsibility to change their ways. There are patients that are feeling less or no pain and want to stop care. They prefer to come back when the pain and disability returns, and they have a relapse.

I strongly advise against the patient stopping care at this point because it only partially corrects the problem. Over time the pain will come back again, and the spine will continue to degenerate because it is still partially out of place making it harder to correct the next time the patient comes back to the clinic.

The patient must be committed to their long-term health at this point. They must be willing to stick with it, make changes at home and improve their lifestyle to get great results. But the ability to do the things the patient loves to do again makes it all worth it!

In this phase I am correcting years of spinal degeneration and breakdown that may continue if the patient and I don't follow through and correct the problem.

The patient is usually coming twice a week when the Corrective Care phase begins. I am flexible with the appointment days and times as long as we get the work done in that time frame. If I recommend twice per week for the next 3 months, then at the next progress exam it is important that we have completed 26 sessions. Each session contributes to the patient's progress and I don't want to fall behind.

During this phase I like to be aware of what may be interfering with the healing process. For example, patients could be under a lot of stress which is causing them to heal slower than a patient with a similar condition and very little stress.

The patient could be eating poorly not giving the body enough nutrition to heal the damaged tissues.

Patients could be overweight and that is putting too much physical strain on the area that is trying to heal.

29 Lifestyle Changes

In the Corrective Phase I will start a discussion with the patient on what they need to do to improve their lifestyle. Quite often the patient needs extra help to make lifestyle changes. They first need to be made aware of the challenges and then a plan must be put in place. Action needs to be taken to make changes and finally there needs to be accountability to complete the changes.

This is where the extra time on the phone can be beneficial. Phone consultations can be a very good way of giving patients instruction and holding them accountable to the work they need to be doing. This can help also to keep the patient on track and, if they are away on business or a holiday, it can serve to prevent relapses.

Changes to a patient's lifestyle can be hard work and difficult. To have a health professional checking in on a regular basis can be very helpful, reinforcing what is needed to make lasting change. This is especially true when that health professional that has your complete history and knows your body well.

The people around you can make a big difference as well. I believe the environment and relationships the patient is in can be conducive to healing or interfere. Support is so important in this phase of healing.

If the patient needs to change their eating habits, then their significant other needs to help by shopping for groceries that will support the changes. Also, when the patient is struggling, they need to give the patient reassurance and encouragement.

Often bad habits develop early in life. The patient most likely emulated their parents and their choices. Also doctors and health authorities only knew so much at the time and some of the recommendations may not have had enough research.

Do you remember when butter was bad for you and now it's good? What we know about health has really changed and evolved over the years. Only 40 years ago smoking was not that bad for you.

30 Nutrition is Important

One of the most frequent recommendations for patients is to improve their nutrition, change their diet, and eat a variety of foods that will help the body to heal.

Nutrition is important to help the healing process in the body because it provides the building blocks for the body to re-build itself. The food the patient eats and what the patient drinks are important for their health and healing.

The old saying "you are what you eat" applies to the patient's body especially when the body is trying to heal. I think there is an extra emphasis during the healing process when the patient is getting adjusted and the body is changing.

I encourage my patients to start reading food labels and knowing exactly what is in their food. They can begin to count calories and see the distribution of carbohydrates, sugars, protein, fats and fiber that are in their foods. I also suggest that patients start to look at the ingredients. What is in the food they are eating? Is it natural and organic? Is the food whole or has it been altered? Are there preservatives and additives in the food?

I like to get patients to investigate the breakdown of the macronutrients in their food. How many grams of protein are they eating? How much water should they be drinking?

How much sugar are they eating? Is the fat they are eating healthy or not?

Patients are surprised how much sugar is in their food. When I started reading labels it seems like everything has sugar added into it! On top of that most foods have modified ingredients, preservatives, colors, and altered fats. I know the products will stay longer on the shelf but are the products good for the patient's health?

I suggest trying to get as many natural and organic foods that a person can get. It is better to eat higher quality foods with better nutrition than buying all the cheapest foods.

I suggest the patient get an app for tracking what they are eating. Some apps allow you to scan the bar code on the food to make input easy. At the end of the day the app will give you a summary of total calories, carbohydrates, proteins, fats and fiber.

The body is constantly evolving and healing. This process is happening every second in a person's body. The body is constantly changing. Nutrition comes in and waste products are going out.

Let's use an example like the spine. The bones in your body are changing all the time and new bone is being laid down called Osteoblasts and old bone is being taken away by osteoclasts. The bones need calcium to be healthy. But if there is not enough calcium in your blood then the calcium is taken out of the bones to be used for more important activities like heart muscle contractions. The brain knows that the heart must beat to keep the patient alive.

There is so much turnover of the cells in the body especially tissues like the skin, hair cells, and red blood cells for example. They have a limited life cycle. Other cells can last longer.

WATER

Water is needed throughout the body as most of the body is made up of 70-80% water. Water allows nutrients to dissolve in it and then transports the nutrients around the body. Water also serves to fill up cells, so they have the right volume.

There is water moving constantly in and out of cells to maintain an equilibrium between the inside of the cell, the outside of the cells and other cells nearby.

Nutrients are needed for cells to be replaced and for new tissue growth. Our diet must keep our body strong and healthy.

Healthy water is water that you would find in nature without any natural contaminants. A good example is water that is fast flowing down a mountain stream that has had time to pick up minerals from the rock bed of the stream along the way. It could also pick up some impurities that could make us sick too.

I like water filtration systems that remove the impurities first but then add back essential nutrients so that the body has the minerals it needs to work well. Personally, I use a Santevia water system to do that. I purchased it at the natural health store in my city. It has a multi stage filter that flows from the reservoir at the top and then when all the water is filtered it sits in a bath of salts and mineral rocks to add that into the drinking water. The water is alkaline. I recommend that patients get a system that is similar.

We are constantly using water to perspire to cool us down, in the urine to get rid of waste, in our stool, and breathing out water vapor from our mouth and lungs. Drinking 8 glasses of water a day has not been proven scientifically so I tell patients that they should drink enough water, so their urine is straw colored. Straw color is a light yellow and when a person gets dehydrated it turns more yellow.

Light yellow urine is a good indication that you are well hydrated. I know this from running many marathons that I want to get well hydrated the day before the race. I stop at all water stations to continue to get water into my system. This will keep my urine as straw-colored as possible but still allow me to sweat out the heat and toxins during the race.

If it gets too yellow, then the urine is an indication that the person is getting dehydrated. Dehydration is not good because the body starts to go into crisis mode to adapt to the lack of water. It affects the way you feel. The body composition is altered.

Clean water with some electrolytes is good for you to replenish the cells. Especially ones in your back that have been damaged and are healing. Nerve cells, muscle cells, ligaments and discs need water and electrolytes to function.

Bottled water may be good or bad depending on the source, the plastic container that it is in and the process to get the water into the container.

Water also serves to carry away toxins and waste products away from the cells. The breakdown of the tissues in the back and the chemicals need to be swept away to provide the right environment for new tissues to come in and heal the back.

ELECTROLYTES

The electrolytes that are dissolved in the water are important too. Sodium, chloride, and potassium are just a few basic ingredients in the cells. The electrolytes help to change the polarity of the cells and allow nutrients to go in and out of the cell membranes with action potentials.

Minerals help to make the body stronger as they provide key ingredients for cellular processes as well. The electrolytes also help the cells conduct electricity and since we are talking about back pain this is important because of the nerve flow traveling through your spine and to the tissues.

We must eat a well-balanced and diversified diet in order to get all the necessary ingredients so the body can function properly. But we must be careful to not eat too much or too many calories can get stored away as fat. It's best to eat foods that have nutrient dense calories that the patient can use for healing and repair.

Empty calories that have little nutrition can lead to weight gain. Gaining weight or being overweight can be bad for the patient's back. It can be stressful. Too much weight can also lead to other health problems like arthritis, diabetes, heart disease and cancer.

The body does need extra nutrition when it is trying to heal. The turnover of the cells and cellular processes are faster and more demanding. The tissues in and around the spine are working to re-build.

A similar process happens when a person gets a cold. The patient may not feel like eating when they have a cold but quickly gets a strong appetite develops as the body begins to heal and needs the nutrition to repair damaged cells.

One of the first things I teach patients about nutrition is to start to eat green leafy vegetables. Green leafy vegetables have many minerals and vitamins that the body needs to re-build the tissue.

Keep in mind that the word vitamin comes from the words vital amine which refers to vital proteins that are necessary for the cells to re-build and function well. Amines are the smaller groups that make up protein. And protein provides the building blocks for the body, like lumber is for a home. These vitamins are proteins that the body cannot do without.

PROTEINS

Proteins serve as the building blocks for the tissues in the back and body. Some of the best sources of proteins come in the form of meat, eggs, fish, tofu, and nuts.

Proteins also help us to feel full, so we don't overeat. Proteins can be converted into energy when there is not enough sugar in the body. I will talk about weight loss later in the book.

I personally think we need to eat more protein earlier in the day to give our bodies the building blocks it needs for the day and to make us feel full, so we don't overeat.

Eating protein earlier in the day is one of the first tips I recommend to patients that want to lose weight. In the typical western diet, we don't eat protein until later in the day around suppertime. But we should be eating protein first thing in the morning to keep the body supplied with the right building blocks for tissue repair.

Without the right supply of protein your body cannot rebuild itself. Bodybuilders know how important protein is for muscle and tissue growth eating protein powder and shakes to build bigger muscles. Patients do not need to go to that extreme eating large amounts of protein, but they need to get enough to allow the tissues to heal.

HEALTHY FATS

Healthy fats are important too and should be eaten earlier in the day. Fats have been unnecessarily given a bad reputation over the past 3-4 decades. Our diets changed to low fat and higher in sugar in the process. Now we are moving back to a healthier balance. Healthy fats are important for our hair and skin. Healthy fats are also important for the cell membranes in our body. Fats are the building blocks for hormones in our body.

A person can get healthy oils from fish, coconuts, olives, and nuts. Healthy fats help the coating of the nerves called myelin. Without the right coating the nerve signals can get short circuited like in the case of multiple sclerosis.

Many foods are promoted as "fat free" which removes the fat and sometimes replaces it making patients think they are doing a good thing for their body. The truth is we need healthy fats, less additives, and a variety of nutrients for our bodies to work to the best of its' ability.

The omega fatty acids are also good for the reduction of inflammation. Also, the brain, spinal cord and nerves need healthy oils to work better. Patients that go on a healthy fat diet like the Keto diet often notice changes to their mental clarity and energy. I think fats serve as a good fuel source for the brain and nervous system.

SUGARS

Sugars are important for energy production. The cells use sugar in the mitochondria to produce adenosine triphosphate which are units of energy that we need to act and get work done inside the body and out.

It is important to stay away from too much sugar and junk food while your body is healing. Sugary treats often lack the vitamins and minerals your body needs and are called "empty calories" for a reason. They provide energy but little nutrients for healing. They can also contribute to weight gain. Also, the insulin spikes from too much sugar can cause a stress reaction in the body. I tell patients to pay attention to the amount of carbohydrates they are eating too. Carbohydrates get converted into glucose in our body. And the less fiber you have in the food the quicker the carbs are converted to glucose in your blood.

FIBER

Fiber is something that the body cannot digest. There are two types of fiber. One type of fiber is insoluble and the other is soluble. Insoluble fiber passes through your digestive system and cannot absorb anything. But soluble fiber can absorb waste products in the digestive system and transport it out of your body.

Fiber keeps your digestive system healthy as it takes up space and cleans the digestive system as it passes through. Fiber also picks up waste products and toxins as it moves through the digestive system and eliminates it.

I like to eat salads to help get enough fiber in my system daily. Fiber also helps to subtract the amount of carbs you are getting from a food. So, if you eat a food with 20 carbs in it but the food has 5 grams of fiber then your net carb amount is 15 grams of net carbs the body will absorb. This is important for low carb diets.

31 Stress

I think stress is one of the most underrated factors in back pain and health in general. I struggled to find books during my career about Back Pain and emotional stress but could see how critical it was in my first couple years of practice. Now I see ads about mental health and how important it is. We have just started to address the issue and we have a long way to go. The awareness of mental health has just started to become something in the mainstream media.

Stress is bad, especially with patients that have back pain because the negative cycle of pain and disability can lead to depression and then poor choices in life. If someone is pre-disposed to depression or mental illness it can be made worse by the back pain. Pain causes chemical changes in the body and the brain.

I do have questions on my intake forms to identify stresses in a person's life and how they are feeling. And as treatment progresses, I want to encourage people to act to make changes to reduce the toxic stress in their lives.

There are certain stressors that patients can do something about and others that patients must learn to accept and have the right frame of mind to deal with. If the mental and emotional challenges are too great for the patient, I will recommend a psychologist or psychiatrist to help.

As doctors we do not have much training on the mental and emotional influences on health and what can be done to help patients deal with those factors when they are present. Most of our study in school was on the physical body, chemistry and how the cells worked. When I went to Chiropractic College stress wasn't discussed much at all.

I did take psychology in premed at the University of Winnipeg and found psychology very interesting. Later when I started practice, I noticed trends in patients that had chronic back pain and were becoming down and depressed.

It was more difficult for them to heal and to make changes that would help the healing process.

I looked for continuing education courses so I could learn more about the psychological aspects of health. And I still look for these types of courses now because I want to learn the latest developments in how patients can better handle their stress.

I believe that we need a lot more education in schools, so doctors are more well prepared to handle patients with significant amounts of stress in their lives. This especially applies to Chronic Back Pain patients.

For example, I really enjoyed going to the Harvard Mind Body Medicine conference years ago. I learned that there was a strong connection between the mind, emotions and the body. I learned how the brain can control different body processes like blood pressure. A patient's mind and emotions could change the physiology of the body! I wanted to tap into that potential so I could teach my patients more. Practices like meditation can be a great benefit to patients to aid healing and deal with stress. Prayer can be just as affective based on other studies.

I now know there is as strong connection between the brain and the healing process in the back. I have seen how stress can produce toxic emotions that can get in the way of the healing process for patients. I could have 2 patients in the clinic with the same condition and one will heal faster than the other because of their stress levels.

I encourage patients to be as real and transparent with their emotions as it will help them to heal. Some patients don't want to talk about their stress at the start of care.

Once some trust is established, they do share their stresses when they feel it is safe. And some never feel comfortable talking about it and hold it inside.

Patients can have stress at work, home, financial stress, or stress at school. I like to know the stress the patient is under to make recommendations for change in the future and better understand the patient. At least to start a conversation to make them more aware of it.

Sometimes it takes a lot of courage to deal with the stressors and to make changes successfully. It can be challenging. But identifying the stressors and making change can be very rewarding especially helping the healing process along and making the body more conducive to healing.

Reducing your bad and toxic stress is important. Toxic stress can come in the form of anger, frustration, and resentment. It can raise the blood pressure, stress hormones, and inflammation in the body. When someone is stressed it causes a fight or flight response which is good temporarily but not long term. The sympathetic nerves start to become very active and then the body goes into hyperactive mode to protect itself and to prepare for battle.

The blood pressure increases to force more blood to the muscles. And the breathing increases to get more oxygen into your system.

Short term stress can be good. I love to run and do half or full marathons. The thoughts, emotions, and physical strain of running a race are temporary. It is something that I want to do short term to accomplish a goal. The training makes me stronger even though it can take a few days to recover from the micro trauma of running. Mentally races can be challenging but I don't do them every day. If I did it would be exhausting and overwhelming! Long term toxic stress can break the body down.

32 Sleep

Sleep is so important for health. I went through a rigorous academic program in Chiropractic College for 4 years. We bragged about how little sleep we had each night. In the early years of my career I worked 12-hour days 6 days a week to help as many patients as I could.

But when I got married and had children, sleep came at a premium. Babies require much attention and when my wife was exhausted, I got up with the babies to feed them, hold them and rock them to sleep. Sometimes that would leave me exhausted. No longer could I keep the same schedule and be healthy. The lack of sleep became counter-productive.

I see this in my patients. Some patients come in with pain that is excruciating. They cannot sleep because of the pain and they toss and turn. The lack of sleep affects the healing process because the brain has circadian rhythms that are important to reset the daily clock in the body. Inside the brain is the master gland called the pituitary. If there is a lack of sleep it affects the nervous and hormonal systems where they meet deep in the brain at the neuro-hormonal axis.

A lack of sleep can cause a downward spiral in the person's health. Patients need relief and rest so the body can focus on repair. When a patient gets their first adjustment the pain starts to go away. For the patient the relief is incredible, and the patient can rest. They are often exhausted from sleepless nights of pain and discomfort. Patients need extra hours of sleep as they get better to catch up on rest.

I have told people that sleep is like a bank account. If there are many withdrawals, then there needs to be deposits to cover the withdrawals eventually or you could go bankrupt in the sleep department. The body is very adaptable but one area where I do find patients have to be very careful is their sleep account which tends to be cumulative.

I often encourage people to take naps to help the healing process. Naps add to the hours of sleep each week. The extra sleep allows the body's nervous system, muscles, ligaments and discs to repair better and faster. The body can focus on one thing while you sleep which is repair and regeneration. It does not have to spend energy on anything else.

I also encourage patients to get in the routine of sleeping at certain times. I recommend a set routine of sleep at certain times each night and waking each day. The body does like to work on an internal clock and routines are very helpful to work with the circadian rhythms.

Also planned naps are good. Patients need to be able to take a break to ease the pain and let the body rest. Even if it's 10-15 minutes lying flat on your back and closing your eyes it can make a huge difference. It does something to reset the rhythms in the brain and aid the healing process. Even if you don't fall asleep, lying down for a nap does provide a mini reset of the patient's brain.

Some people need to listen to quiet music before bed or a favorite podcast. Whatever the patient needs to do to make their environment peaceful will help them to fall asleep. I would recommend a dark room that is slightly cool. And I tell patients not to have any flashing or bright light or chimes going off to prevent the patient from falling asleep or in anticipation of a call or text. Make sure the curtains are drawn to block out any light and the TV is off, so your retina is not stimulated causing you to stay awake. The brain needs some time to ease into the sleep process.

Also, I tell patients that alcohol and caffeine can interrupt sleep or make falling asleep more difficult. So, patients need to be aware of the environment that they are in, get in a comfortable position, and then get the rest their body needs.

33 Mattress

Getting the right mattress is important for back support. Most people sleep 8 hours and they need the proper support for their back.

Generally, I recommend a firm mattress for my patients. The more support the better for the patient's back. If the mattress has coils in it then the higher coil count is best for the back. It seems like the higher coil count keeps the support closer together in the mattress and keeps the patient's spine supported in place. Some of my patients have slept on the floor when they have an episode of back pain and that has provided relief because it is so hard.

I don't recommend memory foam mattresses at the start of care. Memory foam will remember the alignment of the spine but if I am working on correcting the alignment, I don't want the patient's mattress remembering the old alignment from days ago. Later when we correct the alignment of the spine to the maximum improvement, memory foam works great to support the new and proper position of the spine.

If the patient's mattress is old, I recommend they throw it out as soon as possible. I don't want the patient sleeping on a mattress that has poor support as we change the alignment of their spine.

Mattresses need to be rotated and flipped frequently or the support can break down in certain areas faster than others and then not provide the support the patient needs.

A pillow underneath the knees at night helps to keep the pelvis at a better angle and take the pressure off the nerves in the low back. If the patient sleeps on their back one or two pillows under the knees is good. For side sleepers one pillow between the legs is good to keep the hips from twisting.

Sleeping on your stomach is not a good idea. It goes against the natural curves in the spine. You can re-train the way you sleep but it will take time to make that change. I tell patients to stack pillows up on either side to prevent them from rolling over onto their stomach during the night.

34 Core Back Exercises

I have always been a big advocate of physical activity. I have seen the benefits of getting active and staying in shape. I do believe that you must use your body to keep it in shape and to make it stronger. It does not take long to make the body stronger, but it can weaken quickly too. Atrophy can start days to weeks after inactivity. Someone with a back injury that is resting their back is at risk for their back to get weak.

When someone has back pain it is hard to get active. A patient can't do activity because of the pain and disability. One wrong move can cause more pain and set the patient back a few steps.

Chiropractic is great for improving function allowing the patients to use their back more and strengthen their muscles.

Spinal adjustments work to re-align the body. They also work to increase the back's range of motion. Muscles start to change from being tight and protective to be used more for movement so they can relax.

Patients just want to be able to work again, lift their children up, go for walks with their loved ones and do the things they love to do again.

People that have been inactive for a while because of their back pain are prime candidates for some exercise after their first progress exam. Just getting out for a walk may be a good start to getting more active. I liked to encourage patients to use a log or journal to record how far they went and how they felt.

One of the simplest and best activities to begin exercise is walking in a pool. Walking in a pool is great because it provides some resistance from the water but also keeps you more balanced without the fear of falling. It is also better because the buoyancy of the water allows for less compression of the spine especially if the discs are wearing out and the nerves are getting pinched.

I encourage the patient to increase the pace each day and go a little farther. I tell patients to reach for a few hundred yards more and a little faster pace.

Also, a tip that I give patients is to use walking poles if they are feeling like they may be weak or off balance. Pole walking just gives people the re-assurance that they have the support if they need it.

For strengthening it is good to start in the core. There are 4 main muscle layers in the back. Start with the smaller muscle groups adjacent to the spine where the muscles connect one or two vertebrae together.

Gentle movements forward and to the right and left sides can be good for flexibility. I would avoid extending back early in care as it can pinch the nerves and cause spasm. And I would also avoid twisting as it is hard on the discs.

As treatment progresses, I like to advise patients to work with a personal trainer to get stronger. Small coordinated movements can build up strength in the patient's core.

Once that is achieved bigger movements with much more weight can build up more strength in the back. The larger muscle groups travel from the spine to the ribs, pelvis, and leg.

Abdominal crunches can be good to strengthen the front part of the spine but must be balanced with extensions for the back part of the spine. Too much muscle strength in one area like the abs can cause the spine to be pulled forward. The exercises need to be done correctly to prevent injury and to build strength between the segments deep in the core.

That brings me to stretching. I am not a huge fan or doing too much stretching early in care to try to make the muscles looser. I believe the muscles are tense for a reason.

There are two reasons for muscle tension. One is the attachments for the muscles are out of place and the muscle must adapt to the shortened distance. Next the nerve flow is pinched to the muscles and without energy the muscles go into a state of contraction.

Until the underlying condition is corrected the muscles will continue to be tight.

I do like neuromuscular exercises like the wobble board for balance. Reconnecting the nerves, muscles and reflexes is important for balance and healing.

So, it's best to talk to your health professional who knows your back and condition the best to find out the right exercise for you. If you want to talk to me directly please contact me using the information in the back of this book. I would be happy to set up a consultation with you and then talk to your doctor about some of the recommendations in this book that will help you to heal faster, better, and long term.

35 Relapses Can Happen

Relapses are common with Back Pain. I think when the body has been weakened in a spot and has been that way for years it makes it susceptible to re-injury even if that area is rehabilitated. The area may have some scar tissue that makes it weaker and unstable.

I think it is important for the patient to be aware of this and to be extra careful with movements and activities that can re-injure the area. I don't want my patients to walk around scared of doing things but just a little extra cautious with certain activities.

Having said that relapses do occur. The faster we catch a slip, the faster we can get the spine back on track. Patients worry that they have set themselves back to square one when the symptoms return. They feel bad that they may have re-injured themselves after all the work we have done. But I reassure them that we have done a lot of great work to get the area stronger, so a small set back is not the end of the world.

Small set backs are common during treatment. I remind people of this often because I don't want them to have unrealistic expectations about their future and I don't want them to wait to see if the pain will go away without calling me immediately to deal with the shift out of place.

Patients do "fall off the wagon" during care. They forget to do their exercises and may miss visits. In the clinic I encourage the patients to plan. If they know they will be away, I suggest that they make up missed appointments before and after they will be away.

I like to check in with the patient to find out how their stretches are doing. Have they been diligent with the specific exercises I gave them? Are they doing the exercises correctly?

I find the most likely times to fall off the wagon is when the patient travels and they are away from home. Sometimes I find the patient has trouble adapting when they are away to a new schedule and the routine changes.

The change in routine can lead to missed days exercising and a return to old and bad habits. The best way to manage that is to plan and make a schedule including the patient's exercises while away.

Relapses are more common at the start of care when the spine is weak and unstable. They are less common once a lot of work has been done to stabilize the spine. My recommendation is to get checked immediately after any type of slip backward where a patient feels that their spine is not right, or the symptoms are returning.

Also, because the patient has been coming for some time and the spine has been trained to be in a good position again if it slips it will not take much care to quickly correct and re-train it to be back in the right place.

It's like the new position and alignment has become what the body is used to now and the old way is foreign. Before it was the old way that the body was used to, and it took much care and effort to change the pattern. At the beginning of care the spine wanted to go back out of place but now it wants to stay in place.

I think maintaining your care with your Chiropractor is important for long term spinal and overall good health.

36 Weight Loss

Weight loss is so important for the health of the spine, joints and the whole body. More and more people are becoming overweight and obese. This has become a more important topic as more of the population is affected. When I have a patient that is overweight their extra weight works against the healing process because it stresses the joints and there is a greater chance of repetitive strain and injury to the back.

If you have ever been in the gym and lifted weights you know how a 10-pound plate feels to lift. Think about 25 pounds or the biggest plate to put on a bar which is 45 pounds. That is heavy!

And yet if you are 25 pounds overweight you are carrying that weight around your waist each step. The extra weight compresses the bones, joints and discs.

If there are bones already out of place, they are going to wear out faster on one side than the other because of the subluxation but even faster because of the extra weight and workload on the body.

Weight loss is such a difficult subject to approach with patients. It is a pattern that has been there for a long time for most people. Some patients have been overweight since childhood. I was overweight as a child and know that first hand.

There are so many factors involved in being overweight that it can be complicated to lose weight and get in shape especially if you have back pain.

Fat cells grow and divide early in life. They fill up with extra energy from extra calories. As people age and have poor diets that have too many calories not being used the extra calories are converted from glucose to fat to store in our cells

I like to dig a little deeper with the patient to understand when the weight gain started and what were the contributing factors? Is the patient in the right mindset and motivated to lose weight? And does the patient have a support system to make the changes they need to lose weight?

Weight loss can involve a major change in a person's life. It can take a long time to get the changes one is looking for, but weight loss can be very rewarding long term for the patient's spine but also to lower the risk of cancer, heart disease and diabetes.

I have taken courses on Lifestyle Medicine including weight loss. In the past few years I have been educating people mostly about eating habits, physical activity and lifestyle to help them lose weight. Calories do matter and as units of energy if you are not using them the body will store them in the fat cells.

About 3500 calories equals one pound. Simply counting calories can be a good start for most people. And knowing what is in your food is good too.   Reading labels and finding the best food that helps you to achieve a balanced diet with carbs, proteins, fats, and fiber is essential. And mixing up your food choices will give your body a variety of nutrients needed for healing and health. A well-balanced diet will stop cravings and prevent the patient from overeating.

But just counting calories and having a balanced diet may not be enough to lose weight for some people. Some patients need to turn to diets that are low carb to lose weight.

Lately the Keto diet has become popular. Patients are losing weight and getting great results with the Keto diet. My family members have tried it and are feeling better and have lost weight.

There is much information and testimonials on the web and social media about the Keto diet. I encourage my patients to talk to their doctors about their specific condition and any risk factors to the Keto diet. Compared to other types of diets it seems to be one of the more successful ways that patients can lose weight.

37 Prevention and Maintenance

When I initially give a recommendation to a patient, I tell them how much I expect their condition to improve.

Now that the patient's spinal condition has progressed through the Relief and Corrective phases it is time for Prevention and Maintenance.

The patient has made life changes to support their back and they are continuing to exercise, eat better and lose weight.

This is the time when I want to encourage the patient to keep up the changes they have made, keep working to improve, and to keep the check-ups regular.

Check-ups are scheduled anywhere from once a week to once a month in the clinic. This way I can detect any small movements of the spine indicating that it has gone out of place.

The quicker I catch the spine shifting the easier it is to adjust and re-align the segments. The regular visits also give me a chance to talk to the patients about lifestyle habits and what they are doing to improve and maintain their health. I also have an opportunity to hold the patient accountable to some of the changes they have committed to making from previous visits.

I like to stay on top of any new developments in health care that may help the patient. Passing that information on to them about how they can better care for themselves may make their lives even better.

38 Conclusion

Back Pain is very common with 80% of the population having back pain at least once in their life and 40% of the population has it right now. I have seen thousands of patients over my 25-year career that have struggled with chronic back pain.

Patients have tried to cope and do their best with self-care but most often have failed and have become discouraged and sometimes depressed with the pain and disability.

Every patient is unique and needs to be treated that way. A proper history, exam and diagnosis is critical for success. A Care Plan that includes re-examinations, patient education, advice and follow up is important for long term success. Patients need to make lifestyle changes and be supported long term to prevent relapses.

The three phases of care in my clinic are Relief, Correction, and Prevention which includes Maintenance. Progressing through the phases allow the patient to become pain free and get the ability to do the things they love to do again.

I believe educating the patient about their specific condition and what the symptoms mean give the patient a deeper understanding of what they need to do to correct the underlying problem. An educated patient is likely to be more successful at self-care in the future.

The spine and spinal cord are key for a person's health. It is the main highway of communication and electricity from the brain to all the cells, organs and tissues in the body.

Without the proper nerve flow the body is weaker, can get tired and sicker. The sooner subluxations, spinal misalignment and degeneration is caught and corrected the better off the patient will be because it gets harder to treat the longer the body is out of alignment. Wear and tear, degeneration, and arthritis damages the joints and minimizes nerve flow.

But there is hope! Even if other methods have failed Corrective Chiropractic Care and lifestyle changes may be the answer to your long-term health. I encourage you to call a Corrective Chiropractor in your area or contact me for help.

39 Help and advice

If you know someone who has suffered from Back Pain for a long time give them this book. It may give them the information and hope that they need to try something different. Corrective Chiropractic care may be able to correct their back condition and ultimately change their life so they can do the things they love to do again!

If you have Back Pain and have struggled to find a practitioner in your area, please contact me to schedule a Consultation. I will help you find a Corrective Chiropractor in your area that will provide the care I have outlined in this book.

If necessary, I will continue to follow up with the doctor and patient after a referral to help the patient to stay on track during their care and provide lifestyle changes needed for long term results. Sometimes doctors are too busy to provide this service in their clinics and having 2 doctors working together is better than one.

I provide this service through my website www.caryyurkiw.com/consultations. When the reader goes to this page select "Phone Consultation with Dr. Cary Yurkiw, DC".

If you are a doctor and want to improve your results in the clinic treating Back Pain go to www.caryyurkiw.com/practice-management-for-professionals and click "Book an Appointment" and then select "Practice Management Initial Consultation for Doctors and Staff".